The Ageless Path

Harnessing the Spiritual Energies of the Sun

& Raw Egg Yolk for Perpetual Vitality

DexRay

Table of Contents

Introduction: The Path to Eternal Youth

In a world where the pursuit of youth and vitality often feels like chasing an elusive dream, there lies a deeper, more profound truth hidden in the very elements that surround us. This book is not just about health or anti-aging—it's about a journey, one that transcends the physical and delves into the spiritual, the esoteric, and the unseen forces that govern life itself.

Throughout history, humanity has revered the sun as the giver of life, a source of endless energy and renewal. Similarly, the egg has long been seen as the symbol of creation, potential, and rebirth. But what if these symbols are more than mere metaphors? What if they are the keys to unlocking the true fountain of youth—a fountain that flows not with water, but with light, energy, and nourishment that transcends the ordinary?

This book is born from my life, my experiences, and my journey. I do not speak from theory alone, but from a life dedicated to understanding and embodying the principles I now share with you. My diet, my rituals, and my connection to the sun have not only sustained me but have allowed me to thrive in ways that many would find unimaginable.

Here, you will find the esoteric connections between raw egg yolk and the sun—two seemingly simple elements that hold within them the secrets to vitality, youth, and even age reversal. We will explore the profound relationship between cholesterol, testosterone, and Vitamin D3, not just from a scientific standpoint but through the lens of spirituality and ancient wisdom.

You will learn about the sacred practice of naked sun exposure, a ritual that aligns the body with the sun's powerful energies, and how this connection can reverse the aging process and restore youthful vigor. We will dive into the art of mindful eating, elevating it to a level beyond anything you've encountered before—using the mind to fully absorb and utilize the nutrients in raw egg yolk, creating a synergy with the sun's energy that revitalizes every cell in your body.

This book is a revolution in how we understand health, aging, and the very nature of life. It is my attempt to put my stamp on the world, to share with you the insights that have transformed my life and that I believe can transform yours.

As you turn these pages, I invite you to open your mind, to embrace new ideas, and to embark on a journey that could change your life forever. The path to eternal youth is not a fantasy—it is a reality, waiting for you to discover it. And it begins here.

Chapter 1: The Solar Essence of Life

The sun—our nearest star, the source of all life on Earth. Its rays touch everything, giving warmth, light, and energy to all living beings. But beyond the obvious, the sun holds an esoteric significance that has been revered by ancient civilizations, mystics, and seekers of truth for millennia. To truly understand the path to vitality, youth, and longevity, we must first understand the spiritual and energetic role of the sun in our lives.

For as long as I can remember, I have felt a deep, almost inexplicable connection to the sun. Not merely as a source of warmth or a marker of time, but as a living, breathing entity—a force that nourishes my body, mind, and spirit in ways that food alone cannot. This relationship with the sun is not just physical; it is profoundly spiritual. It is this connection that has guided me to the practices and insights I now share with you.

The Sun as the Fountain of Youth

In many cultures, the sun has been revered as the ultimate life-giver, a divine force that embodies the essence of vitality and rejuvenation. The ancient Egyptians worshipped Ra, the sun god, as the ruler of all creation. The Greeks honored Helios, who drove the chariot of the sun across the sky. In Hinduism, the sun is seen as a manifestation of the god Surya, the provider of health and prosperity. These ancient civilizations understood something that modern science is only beginning to grasp: the sun is more than a ball of fire in the sky—it is the very essence of life itself.

But what does this mean for us today? In our quest for youth and vitality, we often overlook the most accessible and powerful tool at our disposal: the sun. Just as plants need sunlight to grow and thrive, so too do our bodies need sunlight to function at their best. The sun's energy is a nutrient in its own right, feeding our bodies with life-giving force that no food or supplement can replace.

In my journey, I have discovered that the sun is, in many ways, the true fountain of youth. Its rays penetrate deep into the skin, stimulating the production of Vitamin D3, a hormone that plays a crucial role in maintaining healthy bones, muscles, and immune function. But beyond its physical benefits, the sun's energy also nourishes our spirit, filling us with a sense of vitality and well-being that is difficult to describe but impossible to ignore.

The Spiritual Significance of the Sun

To fully appreciate the sun's role in our lives, we must look beyond its physical properties and consider its spiritual significance. The sun has always been a symbol of divine power, a representation of the masculine energy that drives creation and sustains life. In esoteric traditions, the sun is often associated with the concept of the "Solar Logos"—a divine intelligence that governs the universe and imparts life to all beings.

This Solar Logos is not just an abstract idea; it is a living presence that we can connect with on a deep, spiritual level. When we expose ourselves to the sun's rays, we are not just absorbing light—we are communing with a higher power, aligning our own energy with the cosmic forces that sustain all of creation. This connection is what gives the sun its rejuvenating power, allowing us to tap into a source of vitality that transcends the physical.

For me, this connection is deeply personal. Every time I step into the sunlight, I feel a profound sense of renewal, as if the sun is infusing me with its life-giving energy. It is a feeling that goes beyond the warmth on my skin or the light in my eyes—it is a spiritual experience, a reminder that I am part of something much greater than myself.

Harnessing the Sun's Energy

Understanding the sun's role as the fountain of youth is one thing, but learning how to harness its energy is another. Over the years, I have developed practices and rituals that allow me to maximize the benefits of sun exposure, both physically and spiritually.

One of the most powerful practices I have adopted is the ritual of naked sun exposure. By allowing my entire body to absorb the sun's rays without any barriers, I am able to fully connect with its energy, drawing in its life-giving force on a cellular level. This practice, though unconventional, has had a profound impact on my health and vitality, allowing me to maintain a level of youthfulness that belies my years.

But beyond the physical benefits, this practice also has a deeply spiritual significance. In shedding my clothes, I am symbolically shedding the layers of ego and attachment that separate me from the divine. I am exposing not just my body, but my soul, to the sun's energy, allowing it to penetrate every aspect of my being and renew me from the inside out.

Of course, naked sun exposure is not the only way to harness the sun's energy. There are many ways to connect with the sun, each with its own unique benefits. Whether it's through meditation, visualization, or simply spending time outdoors, the key is to approach the sun with reverence and intention, recognizing it as the powerful, life-giving force that it is.

The sun is not just a star in the sky—it is the essence of life itself, a divine force that nourishes our bodies, minds, and spirits in ways that go far beyond its physical properties. By understanding and embracing the sun's spiritual significance, we can tap into its rejuvenating power and unlock the secrets to eternal youth and vitality.

In the chapters that follow, we will dig into the profound connections between the sun, raw egg yolk, and the many elements that contribute to health and longevity. But it all begins here, with the recognition that the sun is not just a source of light—it is the very fountain of youth, a wellspring of life-giving energy that is available to us all for FREE, if only we know how to harness it.

Chapter 2: The Golden Elixir— Raw Egg Yolk as a Sacred Food

If the sun is the fountain of youth in the sky, then the egg yolk is its earthly counterpart, a golden orb that holds within it the promise of life, vitality, and renewal. For centuries, eggs have been revered as a symbol of creation and potential, but it is the yolk—the vibrant, sun-colored core—that contains the true essence of this sacred food.

In my own life, raw egg yolk has become much more than just a source of nutrition; it is a cornerstone of my spiritual practice, a daily ritual that connects me to the life-giving forces of nature. As with the sun, my relationship with egg yolk is not merely physical; it is deeply esoteric, rooted in the belief that this golden elixir holds the key to unlocking the secrets of health, longevity, and even age reversal.

The Alchemy of Egg Yolk

To understand the power of raw egg yolk, we must first look at it through the lens of alchemy—the ancient art of transformation that seeks to transmute base substances into gold, both literally and figuratively. In alchemical terms, the egg represents the prima materia, the raw material from which all life springs. The yolk, with its rich golden hue, is the philosopher's stone, the substance that can transform the ordinary into the extraordinary.

From a nutritional standpoint, egg yolk is one of the most complete foods available, packed with essential vitamins, minerals, and fatty acids that are crucial for health. It contains all the nutrients needed to create and sustain life, making it a perfect food in many respects. But beyond its physical properties, egg yolk also carries a profound spiritual significance, representing the potential for renewal and rebirth.

In my practice, consuming raw egg yolk is an alchemical process, a way of transmuting the life force contained within the egg into my own body, mind, and spirit. Each time I consume this golden elixir, I am not just nourishing my body; I am engaging in a sacred ritual, one that connects me to the primordial forces of creation and aligns me with the cosmic energies of the universe.

The Spiritual Energy of Raw Egg Yolk

Just as the sun is a source of spiritual energy, so too is the egg yolk. In many esoteric traditions, the egg is seen as a microcosm of the universe, containing within it the seeds of creation. The yolk, in particular, is believed to hold the concentrated life force of the cosmos, a potent energy that can be harnessed for spiritual growth and transformation.

When I consume raw egg yolk, I am not just ingesting nutrients; I am absorbing the very essence of life itself. This is why it is so important to approach the act of eating with mindfulness and intention. By fully engaging the mind in the process, I can unlock the spiritual energy contained within the yolk and direct it towards my own growth and renewal.

In this way, eating raw egg yolk becomes a form of spiritual practice, a way of aligning myself with the divine forces that govern the universe. It is a reminder that I am not just a physical being, but first I am a spiritual one, connected to the cosmos in ways that go far beyond the material world.

The Synergy Between Sun and Yolk

One of the most profound insights I have gained on this journey is the synergistic relationship between the sun and raw egg yolk. These two seemingly unrelated elements are, in fact, deeply interconnected, both physically and spiritually. Just as the sun nourishes the earth, so too does it nourish the egg, imbuing the yolk with its life-giving energy.

When we consume raw egg yolk, we are not just absorbing the nutrients within it; we are also absorbing the solar energy that the yolk has captured and stored. This is why it is so important to consume yolks that are from pastured, sun-exposed hens—because these yolks contain the highest concentration of this vital solar energy.

This synergy between sun and yolk is one of the keys to unlocking the secrets of health and longevity. By combining the spiritual practice of naked sun exposure with the mindful consumption of raw egg yolk, we can create a powerful alchemical process that rejuvenates the body, mind, and spirit.

The Role of Cholesterol in Health and Spirituality

Cholesterol is often misunderstood and vilified in modern health discourse, but in truth, it is one of the most essential substances in the body. It plays a crucial role in the production of hormones, including testosterone, and is vital for maintaining healthy cell membranes. But beyond its physical importance, cholesterol also has a spiritual significance that is often overlooked.

In esoteric traditions, cholesterol is seen as a carrier of life force, a substance that facilitates the flow of spiritual energy throughout the body. This is why it is so abundant in raw egg yolk—because the yolk is designed to nourish and sustain life. By consuming foods rich in cholesterol, like raw egg yolk, we are not only supporting our physical health but also enhancing our spiritual vitality.

In my experience, the combination of sun exposure and raw egg yolk consumption has had a profound impact on my hormone levels, particularly testosterone. This is no coincidence—both the sun and egg yolk play a crucial role in the body's production of testosterone, a hormone that is essential for maintaining strength, vitality, and youthfulness.

But the effects go beyond the physical. I believe that by supporting the body's natural production of testosterone through these practices, we are also enhancing our connection to the divine masculine energy that the sun represents. This, in turn, helps to balance our spiritual energies, promoting harmony and well-being on all levels.

Raw egg yolk is much more than just a food—it is a sacred elixir, a substance that embodies the life force of the universe and holds the potential for profound transformation. When consumed with mindfulness and intention, it can become a powerful tool for spiritual growth, health, and longevity.

The synergy between the sun and yolk is at the heart of this process, creating an alchemical reaction that rejuvenates the body, mind, and spirit. By embracing this synergy and incorporating it into our daily lives, we can unlock the secrets of youth and vitality and connect with the deeper forces that govern our existence.

In the next chapter, we will discuss the role of Vitamin D3 and testosterone in this process, and how they contribute to the anti-aging and life-enhancing effects of this sacred practice. But for now, remember this: the yolk is not just a nutrient—it is a golden key, a gateway to the mysteries of life, and a powerful ally on the path to eternal youth.

Chapter 3: The Power of Vitamin D3 and Testosterone— Unlocking the Secrets of Vitality

In the quest for eternal youth and vitality, two key players stand out: Vitamin D3 and testosterone. These two substances are often discussed in the context of physical health, but their significance goes much deeper. Together, they form a powerful duo that not only sustains our physical bodies but also connects us to the divine energies that govern life itself. In this chapter, we will dive into the role that Vitamin D3 and testosterone play in the body, mind, and spirit, and how they can be harnessed to unlock the secrets of vitality and longevity.

Vitamin D3: The Sun's Gift to Humanity

Vitamin D3 is often referred to as the "sunshine vitamin" because our bodies produce it in response to sunlight. But this simple description hardly does justice to the profound role that Vitamin D3 plays in our overall well-being. Beyond its well-known benefits for bone health, Vitamin D3 is a master regulator of many bodily functions, from immune response to hormone production. It is, quite literally, the sun's gift to humanity, a vital substance that carries the life-giving energy of the sun into every cell of our bodies.

From an esoteric perspective, Vitamin D3 can be seen as a physical manifestation of the sun's energy within us. When we expose our skin to sunlight, we are not just absorbing ultraviolet rays; we are drawing in the very essence of the sun, transforming it into a substance that nourishes and sustains our bodies on the deepest level. This process is a powerful reminder of our connection to the cosmos, a daily alchemical transformation that aligns us with the rhythms of the universe.

But Vitamin D3's role goes beyond the physical. It is also a key player in the spiritual process of enlightenment. In many spiritual traditions, light is synonymous with knowledge, wisdom, and divine consciousness. By absorbing the sun's light in the form of Vitamin D3, we are not only supporting our physical health but also nurturing our spiritual growth, opening ourselves to higher states of awareness and understanding.

Testosterone: The Hormone of Vitality and Spiritual Strength

Testosterone is often thought of as the "male hormone," but in reality, it plays a crucial role in the health and vitality of both men and women. This powerful hormone is responsible for maintaining muscle mass, bone density, and energy levels, as well as regulating mood and cognitive function. But like Vitamin D3, testosterone's influence extends far beyond the physical realm.

In esoteric traditions, testosterone is associated with the divine masculine energy—a force that embodies strength, courage, and vitality. This energy is not exclusive to men; it is a universal principle that exists within all beings, representing the drive to create, achieve, and overcome obstacles. By supporting healthy testosterone levels through sun exposure and proper nutrition, we are not just enhancing our physical strength; we are also cultivating our inner spiritual power, tapping into the masculine energy that drives us forward on our life's journey.

The production of testosterone is closely linked to Vitamin D3, which is why sun exposure is so crucial for maintaining optimal hormone levels. When we combine the physical practice of sunbathing with the mindful consumption of nutrient-rich foods like raw egg yolk, we create a powerful synergy that supports both our physical health and our spiritual growth. This combination helps to balance the body's energy systems, promoting harmony and well-being on all levels.

The Anti-Aging Connection

One of the most exciting aspects of the synergy between Vitamin D3 and testosterone is its potential for anti-aging. As we age, our bodies naturally produce less of both substances, leading to a decline in energy, strength, and overall vitality. But by harnessing the power of the sun and incorporating nutrient-rich foods into our diets, we can help to slow, and even reverse, the aging process.

From a physical standpoint, maintaining optimal levels of Vitamin D3 and testosterone helps to preserve muscle mass, bone density, and cognitive function—key factors in maintaining youthfulness and vitality. But the benefits go beyond the physical. By supporting these hormones, we are also enhancing our connection to the divine energies that govern life, aligning ourselves with the cosmic forces that sustain youth and vitality.

In esoteric traditions, the process of aging is not just a physical phenomenon; it is also a spiritual one. As we grow older, we are faced with the challenge of maintaining our connection to the divine, of staying aligned with the cosmic energies that give us life. By consciously supporting our bodies with the right nutrients and practices, we can help to preserve this connection, slowing the aging process and maintaining our vitality (forever).

The Role of Mindful Practice

The key to unlocking the full potential of Vitamin D3 and testosterone lies in mindful practice. It is not enough to simply consume the right nutrients or spend time in the sun; we must approach these practices with intention and awareness, recognizing them as sacred rituals that connect us to the divine.

In my own life, I have found that the most powerful way to harness the benefits of Vitamin D3 and testosterone is through a combination of physical and spiritual practices. By meditating in the sun, practicing mindful eating, and engaging in activities that cultivate inner strength and resilience, I am able to align myself with the energies of the universe, drawing in the life force that sustains and rejuvenates me on all levels.

This mindful approach is what sets these practices apart from mere physical health routines. It is the recognition that our bodies are not just physical machines but spiritual vessels, capable of tapping into the infinite energies of the cosmos. By embracing this perspective, we can transform our daily routines into powerful rituals of renewal, unlocking the secrets of vitality and longevity.

Vitamin D3 and testosterone are not just hormones—they are keys to unlocking the secrets of vitality, youth, and spiritual strength. By understanding their role in the body and mind, and by approaching their cultivation with mindfulness and intention, we can tap into the powerful energies of the sun and the cosmos, rejuvenating ourselves on all levels.

The synergy between these two substances is at the heart of the anti-aging process, creating a foundation for health, strength, and spiritual growth that can sustain us throughout our lives. In the next chapter, we will explore the practice of mindful eating at a higher level, and how it can be applied to fully absorb the nutrients in raw egg yolk and sunlight, taking our connection to the cosmos to new heights. But for now, remember this: by embracing the power of Vitamin D3 and testosterone, we are not just supporting our physical health—we are opening ourselves to the infinite potential of the universe, unlocking the secrets of eternal youth and vitality.

Chapter 4: Mindful Eating at a Higher Level—The Esoteric Art of Nutrient Absorption

In a world overflowing with diets, nutritional advice, and superfoods, the true power of eating often gets lost in the noise. We consume food to fuel our bodies, but rarely do we consider the deeper, esoteric connection between what we eat and how it nourishes our soul. This chapter highlights the practice of mindful eating on a level far beyond conventional understanding—an approach where the mind, body, and spirit harmonize to fully absorb the life-giving nutrients of raw egg yolk and sunlight. This is not just eating; it is a sacred ritual, an alchemical process that transforms the act of nourishment into a powerful spiritual practice.

The Sacredness of Food

To begin, we must recognize that food is sacred. Every morsel we consume is a gift from the earth, imbued with the energy of the Universe. The sun's rays nurture the plants, which in turn provide sustenance for animals and humans alike. When we eat, we are not just feeding our bodies; we are participating in a cosmic dance, drawing in the life force that sustains all creation.

Raw egg yolk, in particular, is a potent symbol of this sacredness. It is the concentrated essence of life, containing within it all the nutrients necessary to create and sustain new life. But beyond its physical properties, egg yolk is also a vessel for spiritual energy, a golden elixir that connects us to the divine forces of creation.

To fully tap into the power of raw egg yolk, we must approach it with reverence and mindfulness, recognizing it as a sacred substance that holds the potential for profound transformation. This is where the practice of mindful eating comes into play.

Mindful Eating—The Art of Presence

Mindful eating is not a new concept, but in this context, it takes on a whole new dimension. Traditionally, mindful eating is about being fully present while consuming food—savoring each bite, appreciating the flavors, and eating slowly to allow for better digestion. While these are valuable practices, they represent only the surface of what is possible.

On a higher level, mindful eating involves engaging the mind and spirit in the act of nourishment, transforming it into a sacred ritual. It is about fully aligning with the energy of the food, using the power of intention and consciousness to absorb not just the physical nutrients, but the spiritual essence contained within.

When I consume raw egg yolk daily, I do so with deep awareness and focus, visualizing the golden orb as a source of divine energy. I imagine the yolk's nutrients merging with my own energy field, enhancing my vitality, strength, and spiritual connection. This mental focus amplifies the absorption process, allowing me to draw in the full spectrum of benefits that the yolk has to offer.

The Role of Intention

Intention is the key to unlocking the higher potential of mindful eating. Before consuming raw egg yolk, I take a moment to set my intention, focusing on what I wish to achieve through this sacred act. Whether it is to enhance my physical strength, boost my spiritual energy, or connect more deeply with the cosmic forces, I make sure that my mind is fully aligned with my purpose.

This practice of setting intention is rooted in the belief that the mind has the power to influence the body's processes, directing the flow of energy and nutrients to where they are most needed. By consciously directing my intention, I am able to maximize the benefits of daily raw egg yolk consumption, ensuring that every aspect of its nourishment is fully absorbed and utilized.

This is not just a mental exercise; it is a deeply spiritual practice, one that acknowledges the interconnectedness of all things. The intention I set is not just for my own benefit; it is an expression of gratitude to the earth, the sun, and the universe for the gift of nourishment. In this way, mindful eating becomes an act of communion with the divine, a way of honoring the sacredness of life. It is one of the most enjoyable experiences a person can ever have. Sadly, most will never experience this.

Absorbing the Sun's Nutrients

Just as we can use mindful eating to fully absorb the nutrients of raw egg yolk, we can also apply this practice to our relationship with the sun. The sun is not just a source of light and warmth; it is a living being, a radiant source of life-giving energy that sustains all creation. By approaching the sun with the same reverence and mindfulness that we apply to food, we can tap into its energy in a profound and transformative way.

When I engage in (birthday suite) sun exposure, I do so with full awareness of the sun's power. I visualize its rays gently penetrating my skin, infusing my cells with vitality and life force. I imagine the sun's energy being absorbed into my body as a nutrient, just as essential as any vitamin or mineral. This practice of mindful sunbathing allows me to harness the full spectrum of the sun's benefits, enhancing my physical health, boosting my spiritual energy, and aligning myself with the cosmic rhythms of the Universe.

Naked sun exposure, in particular, is a powerful practice that takes this connection to an even deeper level. By exposing the entire body (even genitals) to the sun's rays, we open ourselves fully to its energy, allowing it to permeate every cell and awaken the life force within. This practice is not just about physical health; it is a spiritual act, a way of connecting with the sun on a soul level and absorbing its divine essence.

The Alchemy of Sun and Yolk

The true power of mindful eating and sun exposure lies in the alchemical synergy between the two. When we combine the sacred practice of consuming raw egg yolk with the mindful absorption of sunlight, we create a powerful process of transformation that enhances both our physical and spiritual well-being.

This alchemy is not just a metaphor; it is a real, tangible process that takes place within the body. The nutrients in raw egg yolk, when combined with the energy of the sun, create a powerful synergy that boosts hormone production, enhances vitality, and supports the body's natural healing processes. But beyond the physical, this alchemy also takes place on a spiritual level, aligning us with the divine forces that govern life and creation.

By practicing mindful eating and sun exposure together, we can unlock the full potential of this alchemical process, creating a state of harmony and balance within ourselves that radiates out into the world. This is the true power of mindful eating on a higher level—a practice that not only nourishes the body but also feeds the soul.

Mindful eating, when practiced at a higher level, becomes a powerful tool for transformation—a way of fully absorbing the life-giving nutrients of raw egg yolk and sunlight, and using them to enhance our physical, mental, and spiritual well-being. This practice is not just about health; it is about aligning ourselves with the divine forces of the universe, creating a state of harmony and balance that supports our journey towards eternal youth and vitality.

In the next chapter, we will discuss the concept of the sun as a nutrient in itself, delving deeper into the esoteric significance of sunlight and its role in the process of rejuvenation and age reversal. But for now, remember this: by approaching food and sunlight with mindfulness and intention, we can transform the simple act of nourishment into a sacred ritual, one that connects us to the divine and unlocks the secrets of vitality and longevity.

Chapter 5: The Sun as a Nutrient—Absorbing the Divine Essence of Light

We often think of nutrients as substances found in food, something we can touch, taste, and digest. But what if I told you that one of the most potent nutrients doesn't come from the ground, but from the sky? The sun, the radiant heart of our solar system, is more than just a source of warmth and light; it is a life-giving force, a nutrient in itself that nourishes not only our bodies but also our souls. In this chapter, we will dive into the concept of the sun as a nutrient, delving into its esoteric significance and the profound ways in which it sustains life, promotes rejuvenation, and connects us to the divine.

The Sun—The Ultimate Source of Life

From the dawn of human civilization, the sun has been revered as a source of life and power. Ancient cultures worshiped the sun as a god, recognizing its central role in sustaining all living things. The sun's rays provide the energy that drives the processes of photosynthesis, enabling plants to grow and produce the oxygen we breathe. Without the sun, life on earth would not exist.

But the sun's influence goes far beyond its physical effects. In esoteric traditions, the sun is seen as a conduit for divine energy, a celestial being that radiates the light of creation throughout the universe. Its rays are not just a source of physical nourishment; they are a manifestation of the cosmic life force, a direct link between the physical and the spiritual realms.

When we expose ourselves to the sun, we are not just soaking up UV rays; we are absorbing the sun's divine essence, taking in its life-giving energy on a cellular and spiritual level. This process of sun absorption is a form of nourishment just as vital as eating food, one that feeds not only our bodies but also our souls.

Sunlight as a Nutrient

The idea of sunlight as a nutrient may seem unconventional, but it is grounded in both science and esoteric wisdom. Physically, sunlight is essential for the production of Vitamin D3, a crucial hormone that supports bone health, immune function, and mood regulation. But the benefits of sunlight go far beyond this.

When we speak of sunlight as a nutrient, we are referring to its ability to nourish us on multiple levels—physical, mental, and spiritual. Just as the body requires food to sustain itself, it also requires sunlight to thrive. The sun's rays penetrate deep into our cells, activating processes that promote healing, rejuvenation, and vitality. This is why cultures around the world have practiced sunbathing and sun worship for millennia, recognizing the sun's power to renew and revitalize.

But sunlight's role as a nutrient is not limited to its physical effects. From an esoteric perspective, sunlight is a carrier of spiritual energy, a nutrient that feeds our souls and aligns us with the cosmic rhythms of the universe. When we consciously absorb sunlight, we are not just fueling our bodies; we are connecting with the divine, drawing in the light of creation and integrating it into our being.

Naked Sun Exposure—A Sacred Practice

One of the most powerful ways to absorb the sun's nutrients is through naked sun exposure. This practice, often overlooked in modern times, is a sacred ritual that allows us to fully connect with the sun's energy, free from the barriers of clothing and societal norms.

Naked sun exposure is about more than just getting a tan; it is a form of communion with the sun, a way of opening ourselves completely to its life-giving rays. When we expose our entire body to the sun, we allow its energy to penetrate every cell, nourishing us on a deep, holistic level. This practice is not just physical; it is also deeply spiritual, a way of aligning ourselves with the sun's divine essence and absorbing its nutrients in their purest form.

In my own life, I have found naked sun exposure to be one of the most powerful practices for maintaining vitality, youth, and spiritual connection. By embracing the sun in its full glory, I am able to draw in its life force, renewing my energy and aligning myself with the cosmic flow. This practice is a daily reminder of my connection to the universe, a way of grounding myself in the divine energies that sustain all life.

The Alchemy of Sunlight and Raw Egg Yolk

As we have discussed in previous chapters, the combination of sunlight and raw egg yolk creates a powerful alchemical process that enhances our physical and spiritual well-being. Just as raw egg yolk is a concentrated source of life, the sun is a concentrated source of energy, and when these two elements are combined, they create a synergy that unlocks the full potential of both.

The nutrients in raw egg yolk, such as cholesterol and healthy fats, work in harmony with the sun's energy to support the production of Vitamin D3 and testosterone, hormones that are essential for maintaining youth, strength, and vitality. But beyond the physical benefits, this combination also creates a powerful spiritual alchemy, one that aligns us with the divine forces of creation and rejuvenation.

When I consume raw egg yolk and engage in sun exposure, I do so with the awareness that I am participating in a sacred ritual, one that nourishes my body, mind, and spirit. I visualize the sun's rays infusing the yolk's nutrients with divine energy, creating a powerful elixir that enhances my vitality and spiritual connection. This practice is not just about health; it is about embracing the full spectrum of life's energies and integrating them into my being.

The Fountain of Youth—Esoteric Rejuvenation

The concept of the Fountain of Youth has fascinated humanity for centuries. While many seek it in physical terms, I believe that the true

Fountain of Youth lies in our connection to the divine energies of the universe. By embracing the sun as a nutrient and practicing mindful eating of raw egg yolk, we can tap into this eternal source of vitality and rejuvenation.

From an esoteric perspective, the Fountain of Youth is not a physical place but a state of being, a condition of perfect harmony with the cosmic forces that govern life. It is a state where the body is fully nourished, the mind is clear, and the spirit is aligned with the divine. This state can be achieved by consciously absorbing the nutrients of the sun and raw egg yolk, creating a powerful synergy that renews and revitalizes us on all levels.

By embracing the practices outlined in this book, we can access the Fountain of Youth within ourselves, unlocking the secrets of eternal vitality and spiritual connection. This is not just a metaphor; it is a real, tangible process that takes place within the body and soul, a process that can be experienced by anyone who is willing to open themselves to the divine energies of the universe.

The sun is not just a distant star; it is a living, breathing entity that nourishes and sustains us on every level. By embracing the sun as a nutrient and integrating its energy into our lives, we can unlock the full potential of our physical and spiritual well-being, tapping into the divine forces that govern life and creation.

In the next chapter, we will delve deeper into the practice of connecting with the sun spiritually, exploring the esoteric rituals and meditations that can enhance our connection to this celestial being and harness its power for rejuvenation and spiritual growth. But for now, remember this: the sun is more than just light and warmth; it is a source of life, a nutrient that feeds our bodies and souls, connecting us to the infinite energy of the cosmos. By embracing this truth, we can transform our lives, accessing the Fountain of Youth and achieving a state of eternal vitality and spiritual connection.

Chapter 6: Spiritual Sunbathing—The Ritual of Cosmic Connection

In our fast-paced, modern world, the simple act of sunbathing has become a rare luxury, often relegated to vacations or times of leisure. But sunbathing, when done with intention and awareness, can be much more than a way to relax or tan our skin. It can become a sacred ritual, a form of communion with the cosmos that rejuvenates the body, mind, and spirit. In this chapter, we will delve into the art of spiritual sunbathing, a practice that transcends the physical and taps into the profound energies of the sun as a source of healing and divine connection.

The Sacred Act of Spiritual Sunbathing

Spiritual sunbathing is not just about lying in the sun; it is about consciously absorbing the sun's rays with a deep awareness of their spiritual significance. It is about opening yourself to the sun's energy, allowing it to penetrate every cell of your body and soul, and integrating its light into your very being.

To engage in spiritual sunbathing, you must first prepare yourself mentally and spiritually. This is not a casual activity, but a sacred ritual that requires intention and focus. Begin by finding a quiet, peaceful space where you can be alone with the sun, free from distractions and interruptions, where you can fully immerse yourself in nature and connect with the earth as well as the sun.

Before you begin, take a moment to center yourself. Close your eyes, take a few deep breaths, and clear your mind of any thoughts or worries. Focus on your breath, allowing it to slow and deepen, grounding yourself in the present moment. As you breathe, visualize yourself surrounded by a warm, golden light, the light of the sun. Imagine this light enveloping you, protecting you, and filling you with its life-giving energy.

The Ritual of Sun Absorption

Once you are centered and focused, you are ready to begin the ritual of sun absorption. Find a comfortable position where you can fully expose your body to the sun's rays. If possible, practice this ritual completely naked, as it allows the sun's energy to penetrate your skin without any barriers. If this is not possible, wear minimal, loose-fitting clothing that allows as much of your skin as possible to be exposed to the sun.

As you lie or sit in the sun, close your eyes and turn your face towards the light. Feel the warmth of the sun on your skin, and allow yourself to relax completely. Let go of any tension in your body, and surrender to the sun's embrace.

As the sun's rays begin to penetrate your skin, focus on the sensation of the light entering your body. Imagine the sun's energy flowing into you, filling you with warmth and light. Visualize this energy moving through your body, from the top of your head to the tips of your toes, infusing every cell with its radiant power.

As you continue to absorb the sun's energy, you may begin to feel a sense of deep relaxation and inner peace. This is the sun's gift to you, a reminder of your connection to the universe and the infinite energy that flows through all of creation. Allow yourself to bask in this feeling, soaking up the sun's light with gratitude and reverence.

Meditation and Visualization

To deepen your connection with the sun during this ritual, you can incorporate meditation and visualization techniques. As you absorb the sun's energy, visualize yourself becoming one with the sun, merging your energy with its radiant light. Imagine that you are not just lying in the sun, but that you are the sun, radiating light and warmth in all directions.

In this state of oneness with the sun, you can begin to meditate on the spiritual significance of this connection. Reflect on the sun as a source of life, a symbol of the divine, and a manifestation of the cosmic energy that sustains the universe. Contemplate the ways in which the sun nourishes not only your body but also your spirit, and how this nourishment connects you to the greater whole of existence.

As you meditate, you may also wish to (whisper) chant (or in your head) repeat affirmations that reinforce your connection to the sun and its energy. Affirmations such as (my personal favorite) "I am one with the sun," "I absorb the light of creation," or "The sun's energy nourishes my body and soul" can help to focus your mind and deepen your spiritual experience.

The Power of Intentionality

One of the most important aspects of spiritual sunbathing is the power of intentionality. The energy you absorb from the sun is not just physical; it is also spiritual, and the way you receive this energy is influenced by your intentions and mindset. When you approach sunbathing as a sacred ritual, with a clear intention to connect with the sun's divine energy, you open yourself to a deeper level of nourishment and healing.

As you practice spiritual sunbathing, be mindful of your thoughts and intentions. Focus on the positive, life-affirming aspects of the sun's energy, and let go of any negativity or fear. Remember that the sun is a source of love and light, and by opening yourself to its energy, you are inviting these qualities into your life.

After the Ritual

After you have finished your sunbathing session, take a few moments to rest and reflect on the experience. Notice how you feel physically, mentally, and spiritually. Do you feel more energized, more peaceful, more connected? Take note of any insights or feelings that arise, and consider how you can integrate this energy into your daily life.

The Transformative Power of Spiritual Sunbathing

The practice of spiritual sunbathing is a powerful tool for transformation, one that can help you to connect with the divine energies of the universe and integrate them into your life. By consciously absorbing the sun's light and energy, you are nourishing not only your body but also your soul, aligning yourself with the cosmic forces that sustain life.

Incorporating spiritual sunbathing into your daily routine can have profound effects on your physical and spiritual well-being. It can help to increase your vitality, promote healing, and enhance your connection to the divine. But perhaps most importantly, it can serve as a reminder of your place in the universe, a reminder that you are a part of something greater, a being of light connected to the infinite energy of the cosmos.

As we continue our journey through the esoteric connections between raw egg yolk, the sun, and the divine, remember that the sun is more than just a source of light and warmth—it is a living, breathing entity that nourishes and sustains us on every level. By embracing the practice of spiritual sunbathing, you can deepen your connection to the sun's energy, transforming your life and aligning yourself with the cosmic rhythms of the universe.

In the next chapter, we will explore the concept of mindful eating on a higher level, applying these esoteric principles to the way we consume food, particularly raw egg yolk. We will delve into the art of absorbing nutrients with the mind, and how this practice can enhance our physical and spiritual well-being. But for now, take a moment to bask in the light of the sun, and remember that you are a being of light, connected to the infinite energy of the cosmos.

Chapter 7: The Fountain of Youth—Esoteric Pathways to Anti-Aging and Age Reversal

Throughout the ages, humanity has sought the secret to eternal youth, the mythical Fountain of Youth that promises a life free from the burden of aging. What if this elusive fountain was not a place but a practice—a combination of spiritual alignment, mindful nourishment, and connection to the Sun? In this chapter, we explore the profound esoteric relationship between raw egg yolk, sunlight, and their transformative power to reverse aging.

The Esoteric Science of Aging

Aging, in the esoteric sense, is not merely the physical process of the body wearing down. It is the disconnection of the spirit from the body's natural life force. Our cells, when fully charged with spiritual energy, have the ability to regenerate indefinitely. But modern life, with its stresses, unnatural diets, and disconnection from nature, leads to a fragmentation of our vital energy, accelerating the aging process.

To understand age reversal, we must first shift our perspective on what aging really is: a spiritual misalignment, a loss of life force, rather than a predetermined biological fate. The key to reversing aging lies in restoring that lost life force, harmonizing the body with its spiritual energy source—of which the Sun and raw egg yolk are potent catalysts.

The Fountain of Youth: Solar Energy and Cellular Regeneration

The Sun is more than a source of warmth or light. It is the cosmic energy of creation itself. When we expose ourselves to sunlight—especially during mindful, intentional moments of naked sun exposure—we absorb not only vitamin D3 but also a profound, energetic life force. This spiritual energy interacts with our cells, revitalizing and regenerating them on a deep, esoteric level.

1. **Naked Sun Exposure and the Healing Light**: The practice of exposing your skin to sunlight without barriers, such as clothing, enhances the body's ability to absorb its full energetic potential. Naked sun exposure symbolizes a return to

nature, an unfiltered connection to the divine source. Every cell in your body is like a solar panel, absorbing and converting this energy into vitality, contributing to the anti-aging process.

2. **Sunlight as a Nutrient**: Nutrients are often thought of as physical substances like vitamins, minerals, and proteins. However, sunlight itself is a nutrient for the spirit and the body. It nourishes the soul in ways that are just as critical as food. When you absorb the Sun's energy, it charges your cells with vitality, promoting not only physical health but also spiritual rejuvenation. This energy is a key component of what keeps us youthful and vibrant.

Raw Egg Yolk: A Gateway to Youth

Raw egg yolk, with its golden hue mirroring the Sun, is a powerful symbol and physical embodiment of life force. It contains essential fats, cholesterol, and nutrients that promote hormonal balance and cellular repair. But beyond its physical benefits, egg yolk is an esoteric substance that, when consumed with spiritual intention, activates deep regenerative processes.

1. **Nutritional and Spiritual Fusion**: The yolk of an egg contains the potential for life itself. When we consume raw egg yolk, we are not just taking in nutrients; we are ingesting pure potential, the essence of life. This potential is what makes egg yolk a powerful anti-aging substance. Its ability

to harmonize with our body's natural energy centers, especially when consumed mindfully, allows us to tap into a deeper, spiritual nourishment that reverses the signs of aging.

2. **Cholesterol and Testosterone as Vital Forces**: Esoterically, cholesterol is the building block of life. It forms the foundation of hormones like testosterone, which governs vitality, strength, and youthfulness. When we consume raw egg yolk, we support our body's natural ability to produce testosterone, the hormone most closely linked to longevity and vitality. Testosterone fuels both physical and spiritual energy, keeping the body strong and the spirit aligned with the source of life.

The Spiritual Power of Mindful Eating for Longevity

Mindful eating is not just a method for better digestion—it is a way to harness the full energetic potential of the foods we consume. By elevating the act of eating into a spiritual practice, we allow the nutrients we consume, like those from raw egg yolk, to be absorbed on a higher level. This deep absorption facilitates the body's ability to heal, regenerate, and maintain youthfulness.

1. **Higher Consciousness and Food**: When you approach your food, especially something as powerful as raw egg yolk, with heightened awareness, you enable your body to extract not only its physical nutrients but also its energetic essence.

Every taste becomes an act of communion with the life force contained within the food, allowing it to nourish your spirit as much as your body.

2. **Absorbing Life Force**: Beyond vitamins and minerals, food carries a vibrational frequency—the life force of nature itself. Raw egg yolk, as a substance that mirrors the Sun, carries this life force in a potent form. By eating mindfully, you amplify your body's ability to absorb this energy. Over time, this spiritual absorption contributes to reversing the aging process, keeping your cells charged with life force.

Harmonizing Solar and Nutritional Energy for Anti-Aging

The true Fountain of Youth lies in the harmony between solar energy and mindful consumption of raw egg yolk. When practiced together, they create a cycle of regeneration and vitality that transcends the limitations of ordinary aging.

1. **Synergy of Sun and Egg Yolk**: The Sun charges the body with life force, while raw egg yolk provides the physical and spiritual building blocks to rejuvenate the body's cells. Together, they form a symbiotic relationship, with each enhancing the effects of the other. The Sun activates the life force within the yolk, and the nutrients within the yolk enhance

the body's ability to absorb and use solar energy.

2. **The Power of Intentions in Youthfulness**: As you engage in both sun exposure and mindful consumption of raw egg yolk, hold clear intentions for anti-aging and regeneration. The mind is a powerful tool in this process. By setting a clear, focused intention on reversing aging and embodying youth, you direct your body's energy to follow suit. With each sunrise, as you stand naked in the light and consume the golden yolk, envision your body's cells regenerating, growing younger, and becoming revitalized.

The Eternal Youth Within You

The Fountain of Youth is not a myth, nor is it something external. It exists within you—activated through spiritual practices, mindful nourishment, and the harmonization of your body's energies with the cosmic forces of the Sun. By integrating these practices into your life, you become the embodiment of agelessness, living proof that aging is not an inevitability but a choice.

This chapter closes with an invitation: embrace the Solar-Yolk connection, and allow the forces of nature to guide you toward a timeless, vibrant life. You hold the keys to your own Fountain of Youth—use them wisely, and age shall become a forgotten concept.

This chapter deepens the spiritual and esoteric connection between the practices you've already established, focusing on anti-aging and age reversal through intentional nourishment and connection to solar energy.

Chapter 8: Mindful Eating—Unlocking the Higher Consciousness of Nutrient Absorption

Eating, in its most basic form, sustains life. Yet, what if I told you that eating could be far more than just a means to survive? What if the very act of consuming food could elevate your consciousness, awaken latent spiritual energies, and unlock the true potential of your body and mind? In this chapter, we'll explore a radical and esoteric approach to nourishment—one that transcends the physical digestion of food and enters the realm of mindful, energetic absorption of nutrients. Here, we move beyond any concept you've encountered before, diving into the sacred practice of eating with full mental and spiritual awareness, where the mind becomes a powerful tool in the digestive process.

The Mind as the Ultimate Digestive Organ

For millennia, humans have viewed the stomach and intestines as the central organs for digestion and nutrient absorption. While this is true on a biological level, from an esoteric standpoint, it is the mind that plays the ultimate role in determining how nutrients are absorbed and utilized by the body. In fact, when you eat mindfully and with conscious intention, you can activate hidden capabilities within yourself that allow you to absorb the full, spiritual essence of food, particularly from raw, nutrient-dense sources like egg yolk.

Egg yolks, especially when consumed raw, are rich in life-giving nutrients such as vitamins, minerals, and healthy fats, but beyond that, they carry a potent life force. This life force can only be fully absorbed when the mind is engaged during the act of eating. To access this deeper layer of nourishment, we must approach eating not as a mechanical action, but as a sacred ritual of communion with the life energies in the food itself.

Eating as a Sacred Act

To harness the power of mindful eating, we must first shift our perception of food. Every time we consume something, we are participating in a sacred exchange with the universe. The food we eat, particularly raw egg yolk, is infused with the energy of the Earth and the Sun. It holds within it the concentrated essence of life. When we eat, we are not just feeding our bodies—we are merging with the energies and spiritual frequencies of the natural world.

To engage in mindful eating, the first step is to recognize this sacred exchange. Set an intention before you eat, acknowledging that the food before you is a gift from the cosmos. Give thanks to the Earth for providing the nutrients and the Sun for infusing the food with its life-giving energy. This simple act of gratitude opens your mind and heart, preparing you to receive the full spectrum of nourishment that the food offers.

The Ritual of Mindful Eating

Once your intention is set, engage in the following ritual for mindful eating, especially when consuming raw egg yolk:

1. **Prepare Your Environment:** Sit in a calm, quiet space, free from distractions. Silence your phone, turn off the television, and create a serene atmosphere that allows you to focus entirely on the experience of eating. Listening to music is great for creating a feeling state that you will over time unconsciously gravitate towards every time that you eat.

2. **Breath and Focus:** Before eating, take several deep, slow breaths. As you breathe, visualize a golden light, similar to the color of the egg yolk, filling your body.

This light represents the cosmic energy of the Sun, merging with your own life force. As you breathe, allow your mind to become fully present.

3. **Attune to the Energy of the Egg Yolk:** Spend a moment observing the yolk closely. Pay attention to the vibrant color of the egg yolk—it mirrors the Sun itself. This is not a coincidence but a spiritual sign of the deep connection between the egg and solar energy. As you gaze upon the yolk, imagine that the energy of the Sun is alive within it, waiting to be absorbed & utilized by you.

4. **Slow and Conscious Consumption:** When you begin eating, do so slowly, savoring every moment. Focus on the

texture, flavor, and sensations of the food. As you chew and swallow, engage your mind fully in the process. Visualize the nutrients from the egg yolk being absorbed directly into your cells, energizing your body at a cellular level.

5. **Mental Absorption of Nutrients:** This is the key to higher-level mindful eating. As you eat, use your mind to direct the nutrients to the areas of your body that need healing, strength, or vitality. For example, if you feel depleted, mentally direct the energy of the egg yolk to your cells, picturing it revitalizing you from within. If you seek to enhance your testosterone levels, visualize the yolk's nutrients stimulating your endocrine system, boosting your hormonal health.

6. **Feel the Energy Exchange:** As you eat, feel the energetic exchange between you and the food. Sense the life force of the egg yolk merging with your own energy. This is not a one-way interaction; you are not simply consuming the yolk, but absorbing its spiritual essence into your being. As you eat, repeat an affirmation such as: "I absorb the essence of life. Nourishing my body, mind, and spirit completely."

The Sun as a Nutrient

In addition to mindful eating, it's essential to acknowledge the Sun as a direct source of nourishment. Just as the egg yolk carries the life force of the Sun, the Sun itself offers a form of spiritual nutrition that we absorb directly through our skin, eyes, and energetic field. This concept takes us beyond the physical absorption of vitamin D3, which the Sun naturally provides, and into the realm of esoteric nutrition.

Much like the nutrients in food, sunlight contains frequencies and energies that are crucial to our overall health. Ancient civilizations revered the Sun as a deity because they understood that it is more than just a star—it is a cosmic source of life energy. In this context, we don't just eat food to stay alive; we also "consume" sunlight, absorbing its energetic properties into our bodies.

Nourishing the Light Body

Our physical body is sustained by food, but our light body—the energetic aspect of our being—

is sustained by solar energy. The Sun emits light codes and frequencies that interact with our light body, activating dormant spiritual potential and aligning us with higher states of consciousness. This is why intentional sun exposure, particularly fully naked sunbathing, is so essential to the practice of mindful eating.

By combining the physical act of mindful eating with regular exposure to the Sun, you can nourish both your physical and energetic bodies, achieving a deeper level of health and vitality. You will not only experience the physical benefits of nutrient absorption and hormonal balance but also spiritual elevation and energetic renewal.

The art of mindful eating is about more than just paying attention to the food you consume—it is about using the mind as a tool to unlock the full potential of the nutrients in that food. By approaching eating as a sacred act and combining it with an awareness of the Sun's energetic nourishment, you can tap into a higher level of consciousness and wellness.

In the next chapter, we will discuss how this heightened state of mind and body can lead to profound transformations in aging, vitality, and even the reversal of the aging process. By integrating these esoteric practices, you are taking a bold step toward reclaiming your connection with the natural world, your spiritual essence, and the eternal energy of the Sun.

Chapter 9: The Esoteric Fountain of Youth—Reversing the Aging Process

Aging has long been viewed as an inevitable process—a slow decline of vitality, energy, and youth. But what if aging isn't the rigid, irreversible process we've been conditioned to believe? What if, through a profound understanding of the mind-body connection, the sun's power, and the spiritual significance of food, we could unlock the secrets to not only slowing down aging but potentially reversing it? This chapter delves deep into the esoteric principles that connect anti-aging and even age reversal with the spiritual practices of mindful eating, sun connection, and the inner power of life-giving elements like raw egg yolk.

Aging as an Illusion of Separation

In the esoteric tradition, aging is often seen not just as a biological process but as a result of our separation from nature's fundamental energies. Over time, as we lose our connection with these elemental forces—such as the Sun, the Earth, and the life energies within food—our bodies begin to reflect that disconnection. The gradual decline we associate with aging stems from this growing gap between our energetic essence and the life-giving forces that surround us.

From this perspective, the key to anti-aging and age reversal lies in reestablishing a harmonious relationship with these powerful energies. When we reconnect with the Sun and the life force within the foods we eat, we realign our bodies with their natural state—one of vitality, regeneration, and youthfulness.

The Sun's Role in Age Reversal

The Sun, long revered by ancient civilizations as a source of divine energy, plays a crucial role in the process of age reversal. As mentioned in earlier chapters, the Sun is more than just a provider of vitamin D3—it is a direct source of life energy that nourishes our body on a cellular and energetic level. It is through regular and intentional exposure to sunlight, particularly in its most natural form (naked sunbathing), that we can tap into this regenerative power.

The practice of naked sun exposure allows for the full absorption of solar energy through the skin, which is not only beneficial for physical health but also essential for reawakening dormant energetic centers within the body. When we expose ourselves fully to the Sun's rays, we are aligning ourselves with its life-giving force, promoting cellular regeneration, boosting hormone production (including testosterone), and activating the body's natural anti-aging mechanisms.

But sunlight does more than just energize the body. Esoterically, it is a key component of the life force, or *prana*, that animates all living beings. When we consciously absorb sunlight with the intention of revitalizing our bodies, we are directing this life force toward rejuvenation and healing. The Sun, as an alchemical source, transforms our cells and energy centers, promoting the regeneration of tissues, increasing vitality, and preserving youth.

Raw Egg Yolk—The Symbol of Eternal Life

Raw egg yolk plays a central role in the esoteric practice of age reversal, serving as both a physical and symbolic representation of life energy. As discussed earlier, the egg yolk is a concentrated source of nutrients, mirroring the Sun in its appearance and energetic properties. When consumed raw, its essence retains its full vitality, which can be harnessed by the body to stimulate the natural regenerative processes.

In esoteric teachings, the egg symbolizes new beginnings, creation, and the potential for eternal life. The yolk, in particular, represents the core of that potential—the concentrated life force that fuels creation. When you consume raw egg yolk, especially in conjunction with solar practices, you are imbibing this life force directly into your body, allowing it to awaken and rejuvenate your cells from within.

By consuming raw egg yolk with mindful awareness, you open the door to its deeper energetic benefits. You activate its life-giving properties in a way that goes beyond mere nutrition, turning it into a tool for renewal and transformation. Paired with the power of the Sun, the raw egg yolk becomes a conduit for age reversal, restoring your body to its optimal state of youth and vitality.

Activating the Body's Regenerative Capacity

Our bodies have an inherent capacity for self-regeneration, but in the modern world, this ability is often diminished due to poor dietary habits, lack of sun exposure, and mental or emotional blockages. However, this capacity can be reignited through the conscious practice of reconnecting with the energies of the Sun and life-sustaining foods like raw egg yolk. When we understand that aging is largely a symptom of separation from these natural forces, we can begin to heal that separation and allow our bodies to repair, regenerate, and thrive.

A key aspect of this practice is the conscious direction of energy. In Chapter 8, we explored how the mind can be used to direct nutrients from food to specific areas of the body. This same principle can be applied to the process of age reversal. By focusing the mind during sun exposure or while eating raw egg yolk, you can direct this regenerative energy toward the cells, tissues, and organs that require renewal.

Imagine the Sun's energy as a golden light that penetrates your body and permeates every cell. As this light enters your body, visualize it repairing damaged tissues, rejuvenating skin cells, and restoring the vitality of your entire system. Similarly, when consuming raw egg yolk, focus on the life force within the yolk merging with your body's own life force, triggering deep, cellular regeneration. By engaging the mind in this way, you are not merely eating or sunbathing—you are practicing a form of energy medicine, using these natural elements to awaken your body's full potential for youthfulness and longevity.

The Fountain of Youth as an Esoteric Concept

In myths and legends, the Fountain of Youth is often depicted as a mystical spring with the power to grant eternal life or restore youth to those who drink from it. Esoterically, this concept can be understood as a metaphor for the life force that exists within and around us, particularly in the Sun, in nature, and in the foods we eat. The true Fountain of Youth is not a physical place but a state of being—one that is achieved through conscious alignment with these life-giving energies.

By embracing the Sun as a source of nourishment, by consuming raw egg yolk as a vehicle for life force, and by practicing mindful absorption of nutrients, we can tap into this

Fountain of Youth. It is not found in an external location but within ourselves—activated by the conscious choices we make and the energies we allow into our lives.

The pursuit of youth and longevity is not about defying nature but about harmonizing with it. When we reconnect with the Sun, with life-sustaining foods, and with the energetic potential of our own minds, we tap into the very source of life itself. In this way, the Fountain of Youth becomes not a distant fantasy but a tangible reality that we can all access through esoteric practices and conscious living.

Age reversal is not a far-fetched dream—it is a possibility that arises from understanding and realigning with the natural, life-sustaining forces that surround us. The Sun, raw egg yolk, and mindful eating are powerful tools in this process, offering a path to not only slowing the aging process but potentially reversing it. When approached with an esoteric mindset, these elements unlock a deeper level of regeneration, allowing us to tap into the very essence of life and youthfulness.

In the next chapter, we will discuss how to integrate all these practices into your daily life, creating a harmonious lifestyle that supports both physical health and spiritual awakening. By consistently embracing the principles of solar connection, mindful eating, and the consumption of life-force-rich foods, you will step into a new paradigm of ageless living—one that honors the body, nourishes the soul, and aligns with the eternal energy of the cosmos.

Chapter 10: Integrating the Practices—Crafting Your Ageless Lifestyle

In the preceding chapters, we've delved deep into the esoteric principles of connecting with the Sun, consuming life-giving foods like raw egg yolk, and practicing mindful eating at a higher level. Now, it's time to bring all of these elements together into a daily practice—a lifestyle that not only nourishes the body but also fuels spiritual growth and personal transformation. This chapter will guide you on how to integrate these practices into your everyday life, allowing you to live in harmony with nature, regenerate your vitality, and create a lasting connection with the life force around you.

Embracing Solar Energy as a Daily Ritual

The Sun is not only the source of life but also a spiritual guide that provides energy for the body and enlightenment for the mind. To harness its full potential, it's important to make sun exposure a conscious and intentional part of your daily routine. This isn't about just spending time outdoors; it's about creating a sacred ritual around connecting with the Sun's energy.

Here's how to make this a daily practice:

1. **Morning Sun Salutation**: Begin each day by exposing your body to the early morning sunlight, preferably during the first hour after sunrise. This is when the Sun's rays are gentle yet powerful, rich with the life force necessary to energize

and awaken your body. Feel its warmth on your skin and allow your body to absorb this energy. Imagine the golden light filling your cells, regenerating and strengthening them.

2. **Naked Sun Exposure**: Whenever possible, engage in full-body sun exposure, as this allows your body to absorb the maximum amount of solar energy. Naked sunbathing for 15-30 minutes (or more) a day is ideal, especially during times when the Sun is not too harsh. Visualize the sunlight seeping into your skin, penetrating deep into your tissues, and igniting the regenerative power within you. This sacred practice helps stimulate the production of vitamin

D3, boosts testosterone, and enhances your vitality.

3. **Solar Meditation**: Integrate solar meditation into your routine by visualizing the Sun's energy entering your body and radiating through your energetic centers. This practice not only revitalizes your physical body but also balances your spiritual energy, opening you up to higher levels of consciousness. Focus on your breathing, and with each inhale, imagine the sunlight nourishing your body, mind, and spirit. With each exhale, release any blockages or negativity that may prevent your body from fully absorbing this life force.

The Art of Consuming Raw Egg Yolk as a Spiritual Practice

Consuming raw egg yolk is far more than a nutritional choice—it is a sacred act of ingesting life force. As we've discussed, the raw egg yolk contains the essence of life, and when consumed mindfully, it has the power to nourish your body and soul on a profound level.

Here's how to elevate the simple act of eating into a spiritual experience:

1. **Setting an Intention**: Before consuming raw egg yolk, take a moment to set an intention for what you wish to gain from this sacred food. Hold the egg in your hand, acknowledging the life force it contains. Whether it's enhanced vitality,

healing, or spiritual growth, visualize the nutrients in the yolk becoming one with your body, energizing your cells and activating your inner power.

2. **Mindful Consumption**: Practice mindful eating by savoring the experience of consuming raw egg yolk. Focus on the texture, the taste, and the sensation as it enters your body. With each swallow, visualize the life force of the yolk merging with your own, nourishing every cell and sparking a process of regeneration within you. Envision the yolk's nutrients traveling to areas of your body that need healing or revitalization, using the power of your mind to direct its energy where it is needed most.

3. **Ritualistic Eating**: Make the consumption of raw egg yolk a daily ritual. Combine it with your solar meditation or sun exposure for a full energetic alignment. The egg yolk and the Sun work in tandem, with the Sun's energy activating and enhancing the life force within the yolk. Eating with this level of mindfulness transforms a simple meal into a spiritual practice that fuels your physical and spiritual evolution.

Higher-Level Mindful Eating

The process of mindful eating, as we've explored, goes beyond simply being aware of what you're eating. It involves tapping into a higher level of consciousness to fully absorb and integrate the nutrients you consume. In this section, we will explore advanced techniques for taking mindful eating to a transformative level, applying esoteric principles to extract the maximum life force from your food.

1. **Energetic Alignment**: Before eating, take a moment to align your energy with the food in front of you. This can be done through a brief meditation, where you acknowledge the source of the food and its life-giving properties. As you eat, maintain a sense of gratitude and awareness, recognizing that the food is more than just fuel—it is a part of the cosmic life force that sustains all living beings. By aligning your energy with the food, you allow your body to absorb not

just its physical nutrients but also its energetic essence.

2. **Mind Over Matter**: Practice the technique of mentally directing nutrients to specific areas of your body. As you chew or swallow, imagine the nutrients from the food traveling through your bloodstream and into the areas that need rejuvenation or healing. Whether it's your skin, muscles, organs, or energetic centers, use the power of your mind to focus the nutrients where they are needed most. This conscious direction of energy helps enhance the body's natural processes of regeneration and renewal.

3. **Absorbing the Subtle Energies**: Food carries more than just physical nutrients—

it contains subtle energies that are often overlooked in traditional nutritional science. By practicing mindful eating at a higher level, you can train your body to absorb these subtle energies. This requires deep concentration and awareness of how the food interacts with your body on an energetic level. Over time, you will become more attuned to the energy of different foods, allowing you to choose those that resonate most with your body's needs.

Making the Sun a Nutrient

Just as the food we eat sustains us physically, the Sun sustains us energetically. One of the most revolutionary concepts in this lifestyle is understanding that the Sun is a nutrient in itself. We don't just benefit from the vitamin D it helps produce; we absorb the Sun's energy directly, just as we absorb nutrients from food.

1. **Solar Absorption**: To absorb the Sun as a nutrient, it's essential to cultivate an awareness of how your body interacts with sunlight. Practice visualizing the Sun's rays entering your body and nourishing you from within. Imagine that the sunlight is a liquid golden energy that seeps into your skin and penetrates deep into your cells. By mentally acknowledging the Sun as a nutrient, you enhance your body's ability to absorb and utilize this energy on both a physical and spiritual level.

2. **Sunlight as Prana**: In esoteric traditions, the Sun is seen as a source of *prana*, or life force energy. Just as you absorb nutrients from the foods you eat, you can absorb *prana* from sunlight. This requires an open, receptive mindset and a deep connection with the Sun's energy. When you practice sunbathing or solar meditation, focus on breathing in this *prana*, allowing it to energize and replenish you. Over time, your body will learn to rely on the Sun as a source of nourishment, reducing your dependence on physical food.

3. **Solar Fasting**: As your connection with the Sun deepens, you may find that your need for physical food decreases. This is a natural result of absorbing more of the

Sun's life force energy. Some esoteric practitioners engage in periods of solar fasting, where they consume minimal food and rely primarily on sunlight for energy. While this practice is advanced and requires careful preparation, it highlights the profound potential of solar energy as a nutrient source.

Designing Your Ageless Lifestyle

Bringing all of these elements together—sun exposure, raw egg yolk consumption, and higher-level mindful eating—creates a lifestyle that supports both physical health and spiritual growth. The key is consistency and intentionality. By making these practices a regular part of your daily routine, you will begin to experience the transformative effects of aligning with the natural forces that sustain life.

Your ageless lifestyle is not just about avoiding aging—it's about fully embracing life's energy and allowing it to flow through you, rejuvenating your body, mind, and spirit. With each sunrise, with each mindful bite of food, you are engaging in a sacred exchange with the cosmos (whether you realize it or not), inviting the eternal life force to nourish and sustain you. The more aware of this that you are, the more potential you have for achieving anything that your heart desires.

In the next chapter, we will explore the deeper spiritual implications of this lifestyle, and how living in alignment with these principles can awaken higher levels of consciousness, purpose, and enlightenment. Through the physical practices of solar connection and mindful nourishment, you are opening the door to a much deeper journey of self-discovery and cosmic unity.

Chapter 11: Awakening the Spirit—The Path to Higher Consciousness

As we approach the final layers of this transformative journey, it becomes clear that the practices we've embraced—solar connection, mindful eating, and the consumption of raw egg yolk—are not just physical. They are, in essence, doorways to a much deeper spiritual reality. This chapter will take you beyond the realm of the body and into the realm of the soul, where the ultimate goal is not just health, longevity, or vitality, but the awakening of a higher consciousness.

To truly thrive, we must acknowledge the interconnectedness of our physical bodies with the subtle energy fields and the universal life force that permeates all of existence. In this chapter, we will discuss how the practices introduced throughout this book can be used to awaken your spiritual potential, elevate your consciousness, and align you with the cosmic rhythms that guide our evolution.

The Solar Connection as a Portal to the Divine

Since ancient times, the Sun has been revered as a symbol of divine power and cosmic order. Many cultures believed that the Sun was a physical manifestation of a higher intelligence, a source of life and wisdom. By connecting with the Sun in the ways we've discussed, we're not just absorbing light and energy—we are tapping into the deeper spiritual forces that the Sun represents.

Here's how you can elevate your solar practice to facilitate spiritual awakening:

1. **Sun (Sky) Gazing and Spiritual Clarity**: Sun gazing (NEVER STARE DIRECTLY INTO THE SUN), particularly during the first hour after sunrise and the last hour before sunset, can help unlock higher levels of spiritual clarity. As you gaze into the sky away from the Sun, allow your mind to still and open to the cosmic information that the Sun is transmitting. This practice not only stimulates the pineal gland, often referred to as the "seat of the soul," but also clears mental clutter and awakens your higher faculties of intuition and insight. Begin with a few seconds or minutes at a time, and gradually increase the duration as your

body becomes accustomed to the practice. Lying down on your back for this really enhances the meditative experience.

2. **The Sun as a Guide**: View the Sun as more than just a source of physical nourishment—see it as a spiritual guide that connects you to the divine. The energy you receive from the Sun is both a physical and metaphysical force. By building a consistent relationship with the Sun, you open yourself to receiving spiritual wisdom, guidance, and higher understanding. Allow the Sun's rays to not only energize your body but also illuminate your mind and heart, clearing the way for spiritual growth.

3. **Channeling Solar Energy into Your Spiritual Practice**: During meditation or spiritual rituals, you can consciously channel solar energy into your practice. Visualize the Sun's rays entering your body, energizing your spiritual centers (chakras), and aligning you with higher states of awareness. This practice will heighten your ability to perceive the subtle realities of existence, helping you to transcend the limitations of the material world and tap into the infinite source of divine energy.

Mindful Eating as a Path to Higher Awareness

While mindful eating has powerful physical benefits, it also has the potential to awaken higher levels of spiritual consciousness. By practicing mindful eating with the raw egg yolk, you are not just nourishing your body but feeding your soul. Every mindful bite becomes an act of communion with the life force, opening you to deeper levels of spiritual awareness.

Here are some ways to elevate mindful eating into a spiritual practice:

1. **Energetic Awareness During Eating**: As you eat mindfully, begin to tune into the energetic qualities of your food. For example, with the raw egg yolk, visualize the life force within the yolk transferring into your body, not just as physical nutrients but as spiritual energy. Feel the warmth, the vibrancy, and the subtle

energetic waves as they enter your being. Recognize that food is more than just physical matter—it carries the energetic signature of life itself.

2. **Mindful Eating as a Meditation**: Transform your meals into a form of meditation. Focus entirely on the act of eating, savoring each bite, each flavor, each texture. As you do this, allow your mind to become fully present. This mindfulness opens the door to higher awareness, as it tunes you into the present moment, where spiritual insight often emerges. When eating becomes a meditation, your body, mind, and spirit harmonize, creating an inner alignment that facilitates spiritual awakening.

3. **Connection to the Cosmos through Food**: The raw egg yolk, in its form and essence, mirrors the Sun—the great cosmic life force. By consuming this sacred food with a heightened awareness of its spiritual significance, you are participating in a greater cosmic exchange. The life force within the yolk connects you with the life force of the universe, nourishing not only your body but your spiritual essence. This practice allows you to transcend the physical realm and tap into the universal consciousness.

The Sacred Balance of Masculine and Feminine Energies

Another esoteric concept that becomes clear as you engage in these practices is the balance of masculine and feminine energies within and around you. The Sun, often viewed as a masculine force, provides the yang energy—life, light, and activity—while the egg yolk, a symbol of potential life and nourishment, embodies yin, the feminine energy of receptivity and nurturing.

By integrating these two forces—through sun exposure and the mindful consumption of raw egg yolk—you are creating an internal balance of energies that supports not only physical vitality but also spiritual wholeness. This balance is essential for personal transformation and awakening higher consciousness. Here's how to maintain this sacred balance:

1. **Honoring Both Energies**: Acknowledge the interplay of masculine and feminine

energies within you. The Sun fuels your outward expression, your drive, and your vitality, while the egg yolk nurtures your inner being, providing the foundation for life. By honoring and balancing both energies, you create an internal harmony that supports spiritual growth.

2. **Daily Practices to Balance Energy**: To maintain this balance, incorporate practices that honor both energies. Spend time in the Sun, allowing its masculine energy to invigorate you. At the same time, engage in nurturing practices, such as mindful eating, meditation, or introspection, to cultivate your feminine energy. This balance helps to awaken and integrate all aspects of your being, leading to a more holistic and fulfilling life.

Awakening to the Higher Self

As you continue on this journey, the ultimate goal is not just physical rejuvenation or increased vitality—it is the awakening of your higher self. The higher self is the aspect of you that is connected to the divine, the part of you that transcends the material world and exists in the realm of infinite consciousness. Through the practices in this book, you are cultivating the physical and spiritual foundation necessary to connect with this higher aspect of yourself.

Here are some final thoughts on how to awaken and integrate your higher self:

1. **Recognizing the Higher Self**: The higher self is always present within you, guiding you, and providing wisdom and insight. To awaken this connection, cultivate

practices that bring you into alignment with your soul's purpose. Solar meditation, mindful eating, and daily spiritual reflection are all tools to help you attune to the presence of your higher self. As you deepen your connection to the Sun and the life force, you will find that your higher self naturally begins to emerge and guide you on your path.

2. **Living from a Place of Higher Consciousness**: As your higher self becomes more integrated into your daily life, you will begin to live from a place of higher consciousness. This means making decisions from a place of clarity, compassion, and alignment with your soul's purpose. Your connection with the Sun and your mindful eating practices will

serve as a foundation for this new way of being, providing you with the energy, insight, and balance to navigate life from a place of wisdom and spiritual growth.

3. **Embodying Your Spiritual Truth**: Ultimately, the goal of this journey is to embody your spiritual truth in all aspects of your life. Whether it's through your physical practices, your relationships, or your inner work, you are awakening to a deeper understanding of who you are and your place in the universe. This realization brings with it a profound sense of peace, purpose, and joy, as you begin to live in harmony with the cosmic forces that guide all of existence.

Becoming a Vessel for the Divine

This journey of solar connection, mindful nourishment, and spiritual awakening is not just a personal one—it is a cosmic journey. As you integrate these practices into your life, you become a vessel for the divine, a living expression of the life force that flows through the universe. Your body becomes a temple, your mind a tool for higher awareness, and your spirit a reflection of the eternal truth.

In awakening to this higher state of consciousness, you are not only reclaiming your vitality and longevity but also stepping into your true power as a spiritual being. This is the path to the ageless, the timeless, and the infinite. It is the path to becoming one with the universe, a co-creator of your reality, and a beacon of light for others.

Now, the journey is yours to continue. Embrace these practices, live with intention, and let the light of the Sun and the wisdom of the cosmos guide you on the path to higher consciousness. You are a divine being, filled with infinite potential—let that truth shine through every aspect of your life.

Chapter 12: Manifesting Your Divine Purpose—Living in Alignment

As we conclude this transformative journey, it's essential to understand that integrating these esoteric practices into your daily life is not just about personal growth; it's about living in alignment with your divine purpose. This chapter will explore how to harness the insights gained throughout this book to manifest your highest potential and align with your soul's true calling.

Discovering Your Divine Purpose

Your divine purpose is the unique role you are meant to play in the grand scheme of existence. It is the expression of your soul's deepest desires and the contribution you are destined to make in the world. By aligning with the practices of solar connection, mindful eating, and spiritual awareness, you are preparing yourself to discover and live out this purpose.

1. **Inner Reflection and Clarity**: Begin by engaging in deep inner reflection to uncover your divine purpose. This involves quieting your mind and listening to your inner voice. Spend time in meditation, contemplating your passions, values, and the areas where you feel a deep sense of fulfillment. As you practice solar meditation and mindful eating, allow these experiences to provide clarity and insight into your true calling. Your heightened awareness will guide you

toward understanding how you can best serve your purpose.

2. **Aligning with Your Higher Self**: The practices we've discussed throughout this book—connecting with the Sun, consuming raw egg yolk, and practicing mindful eating—serve to elevate your consciousness and align you with your higher self. This alignment is crucial for manifesting your divine purpose. As you cultivate a deeper connection with your higher self, you will begin to receive guidance and inspiration that will lead you toward fulfilling your soul's mission.

3. **Embracing Your Unique Gifts**: Each person has unique gifts and talents that are meant to be shared with the world.

Reflect on the skills, passions, and experiences that make you unique. How can you use these gifts to contribute to the greater good? The clarity gained from your spiritual practices will help you recognize and embrace these gifts, enabling you to express them in a way that aligns with your divine purpose.

Living in Alignment with Your Purpose

Once you have a clear sense of your divine purpose, the next step is to align your daily life with this purpose. This requires intentionality and commitment, ensuring that every action, decision, and thought supports your soul's mission.

1. **Setting Intentions and Goals**: Create specific intentions and goals that reflect

your divine purpose. These goals should be aligned with your higher self and the contributions you wish to make. For example, if your purpose involves helping others through holistic health, set goals that allow you to develop and share your knowledge in this area. Write down these goals, and review them regularly to stay focused and motivated.

2. **Creating a Purposeful Routine**: Design a daily routine that supports your alignment with your divine purpose. Incorporate practices that nurture your body, mind, and spirit, such as sun exposure, mindful eating, and spiritual meditation. By embedding these practices into your daily life, you create a foundation that supports your purpose

and keeps you in alignment with your highest self.

3. **Living with Integrity**: Aligning with your divine purpose requires living with integrity and authenticity. Make decisions that are true to your values and purpose, and act in ways that reflect your highest intentions. This may involve setting boundaries, making changes in your relationships, or pursuing new opportunities that resonate with your soul's mission. Living with integrity ensures that your actions are in harmony with your true self.

Manifesting Your Vision

With clarity on your divine purpose and a routine that supports it, you are now ready to manifest your vision. Manifestation involves bringing your dreams and intentions into reality by aligning your actions with your desires.

1. **Visualizing Your Success**: Use visualization techniques to imagine yourself living out your divine purpose. Picture yourself achieving your goals, making a positive impact, and experiencing fulfillment. Visualization helps to align your subconscious mind with your conscious desires, creating a powerful force for manifestation. Practice visualization regularly, especially in conjunction with your solar and mindful eating practices.

2. **Taking Inspired Action**: Manifestation requires more than just visualization; it involves taking inspired action. Act on the insights and guidance you receive from your higher self. Follow opportunities that align with your purpose, and be open to taking bold steps that move you closer to your goals. Trust in the process and remain committed to your path, knowing that each action you take is a step toward fulfilling your divine mission.

3. **Cultivating Patience and Trust**: Manifestation is a journey that requires patience and trust. There may be times when progress seems slow or obstacles arise, but trust that you are on the right path. Maintain faith in your purpose and the process of manifestation. Your

dedication and persistence will eventually lead to the realization of your vision.

Nurturing Your Spiritual Growth

As you live in alignment with your divine purpose, it's essential to continue nurturing your spiritual growth. This ongoing practice ensures that you remain connected to your higher self and stay open to new insights and guidance.

1. **Continued Spiritual Practices**: Maintain your spiritual practices, such as solar meditation, mindful eating, and inner reflection. These practices will keep you connected to your higher self and support your ongoing spiritual growth. Explore new practices that resonate with you and enhance your connection to the divine.

2. **Seeking Spiritual Community**: Engage with a spiritual community that shares your values and supports your journey. Being part of a community provides encouragement, inspiration, and opportunities for growth. It also allows you to share your experiences and learn from others who are on a similar path.

3. **Embracing Lifelong Learning**: Spiritual growth is a lifelong journey. Embrace opportunities for learning and personal development. Stay curious and open to new experiences that expand your understanding and deepen your connection to your divine purpose.

Conclusion: Living Your Legacy

As you align with your divine purpose and manifest your vision, you are creating a legacy that reflects your highest self. This legacy is not just about the impact you make in the world; it is also about the way you live your life with authenticity, purpose, and spiritual awareness. By living in alignment with your divine purpose, you contribute to the greater good and leave a lasting mark on the world.

Remember, your journey is a reflection of your inner truth and the divine essence within you. Embrace each moment as an opportunity to grow, to connect, and to live fully. Your divine purpose is a guiding light that leads you to a life of fulfillment, joy, and spiritual enlightenment. As you continue on this path, may you shine brightly, embodying the essence of your true self and inspiring others to do the same.

This is your time to shine, to live in alignment with your soul's mission, and to make a profound impact on the world. Embrace your journey, honor your divine purpose, and let your light guide you toward a future of limitless possibilities.

My 175 lb Weight Loss Transformation

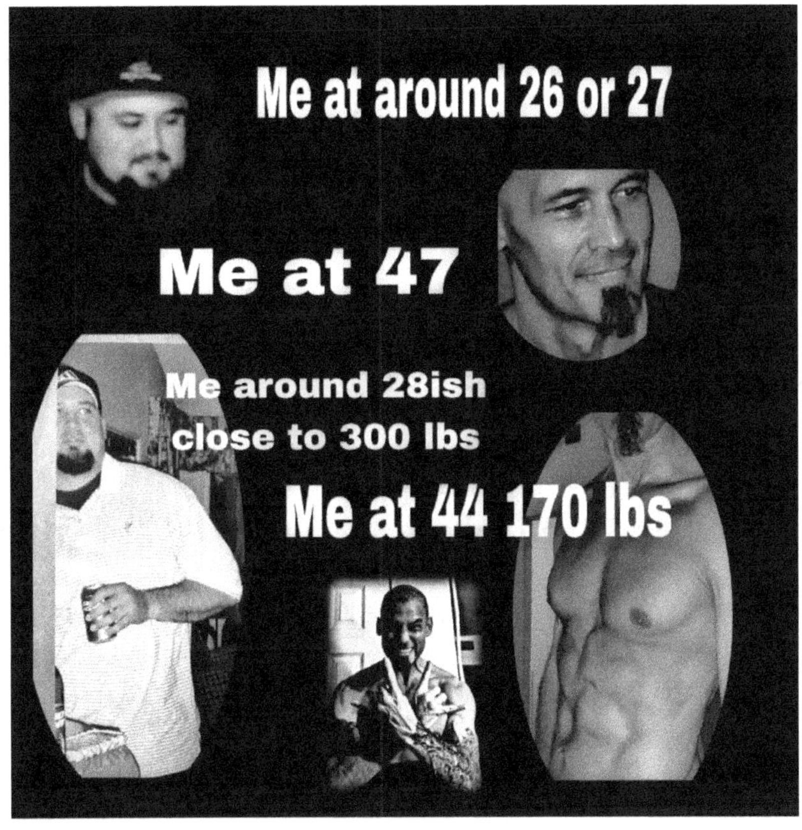

Hey, nice to meet you! I am so thrilled that you are about to dive into my book - ***The Ageless Path***. It truly means the world to me. I have been honing what I call Diet – Lifestyle –

Mindset Mastery, since transforming myself into a brand new ME over 15 years ago as I turned into my 30's. I was born in 1977, & am currently 47 years of age as I write this book - The 1st book in my DLM Mastery Series. About 15 years ago or so I had created a Facebook group that quickly grew to about 20k followers. I eventually shut it down due to the toxicity of negative trolls flooding the group. In this group I was sharing all of my trials & errors (there were many of them) in my quest to attain Diet – Lifestyle – Mindset Mastery. Which started as one of my many mantra's I created for myself to use as fuel to transform myself into what I have become today, & what I intend on becoming in the future. I have no limits to my growth potential. I'm a lifelong student of life itself, forever dedicated to my own journey. I remember telling people (especially the troll's) in my group to wait until I am 50. Just wait until I am 50, & I will have this down, & share it with the world, I would say like a Parrot. I knew way back then that I was onto something special. I just didn't have all of the answers to my questions all lined up in my head correctly. I still don't, & who knows if I ever will. But what I do know is that I will never stop my quest for optimal vitality (it actually goes much deeper than just that). So here I am just a few years shy of a half a century (my earth age) & feeling like a Prime Thoroughbred that never ages. I just could not wait until 50 to begin sharing this with the world. It is time now to begin sharing all of my cockamamie beliefs about life & vitality with the world. I have written some short books, & created countless amounts of videos about my personal transformation that opened up my mind to all of this (& more) I write about in this book. When I was 40 or 41 years old I wrote a book titled – ***How I Lost 100 Pounds in 100 Days***. I had drunk myself to a whopping 330 pounds by the end of my 20's. These pictures right here don't even give you the slightest clue to how bad I looked & felt. I have ZERO pictures of myself at 330 lbs. ZERO! You are going to have to take my word for it. I only have a few pictures of me over 250 lbs. And the worst of the worst looking picture of me is actually my drivers license ID photo, which is on the cover of this book –

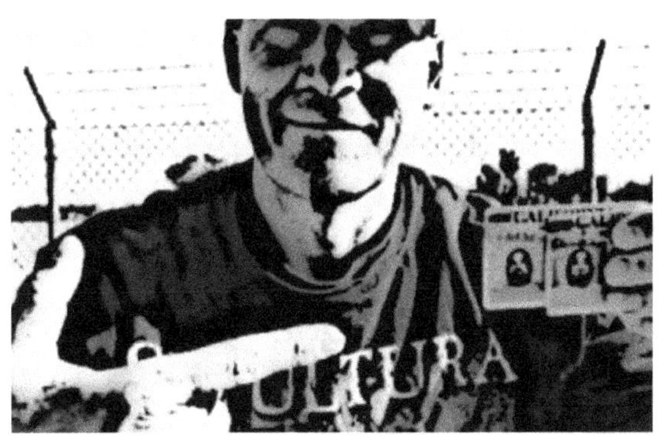

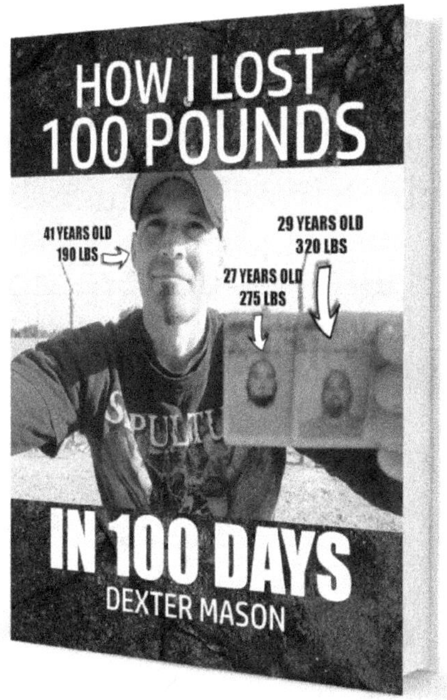

I was drinking a 30 pack a day in order to just remain even keel. On days I didn't have to work, I would add in hard liquor, wine, & even stronger by volume types of beer. I drank daily for over a decade. It began with about a 12 pack a day for my issue, and just ramped up to something that many people understandably find not believable for any one human to consume. I understand that. It sounds impossible to be that much of a lush. Had I not been one myself, I might even not believe it could happen as well. But I lived the lush life for many years. And sadly so do probably millions of other individuals all over this world. I had major demons inside of me that I was trying to drown out. Let me tell you from experience – demons can breathe just fine under water (or alcohol). They might even prefer to work under those conditions. I ended up finding homeostasis in the 190's & felt amazing again as I did as a youth. I kept my weight there up until I turned 44, when I decided to lose even more bodyweight. I did not want to enter into my 50's close to 200 lbs. My instincts are really good when it comes to my own longevity now days. Every ideas and theory I have come up with pertaining to longevity has all came from within me. I have had all these ideas just sprout & eventually blossom into something that contributes to the leveling up of self (Vibe Higher). So at 44 years of age I made the decision to never weigh over 180 lbs again in my life. I am 5 foot 11. But once I got myself down into the 170's, I was feeling so amazing, I decided to see how low I could go, and where I would really be at my best weight wise. So I went down under 170 into the 160's, and even dabble into the upper 150's occasionally for splits & giggles. But my favorite new weight to roam around in is in the 160's for sure. I just weighed myself this morning & weighed 157.8. I have fun with the 150's from time to time, but I have found a really good weight for myself in the 160's all year round. I feel amazing in the 190's. But I feel invincible in the 160's. So if 330 lbs was my heaviest (that I know of) weight. And 155 was the lowest weight I have seen on a scale after 44. Technically I can bull horn shout that I lost literally 175 lbs! That is insane! But I don't ever say it, or think of it that way. I never have. I am not obese by nature. I drank myself to that weight. Poor food choices along with thousands of beer calories a day will eventually catch up to even the best of the best genetics. I have pretty decent genetics. I don't have loose skin, or any stretch marks from being that overweight. I have stretch marks from years of lifting weights since about

10 years old or so. I didn't even have love handles at 330 lbs. I had a huge gut up front yes. But no love handles or saggy fat. Don't get me wrong. I am not taking anything away from my accomplishment. I just know there are people out there with real weight issues that are hereditary. And if that is you, I support you in whatever you need to do to achieve your weight loss & longevity goals. I have actually over time grown to understand that my own personal weight loss story can be very motivational & inspirational to anyone looking to better themselves in general - whether they need to lose weight or not. For years I did not think like this. I was clinging onto some weird type of shame for not being genetically obese. As if I did not earn the right to inspire people with not just my weight loss journey, but my

entire transformation of myself that has no ending to it. That is so weird right? I used to go out of my way to not share my weight loss story with anyone for years. I would never reveal to people what my actual stats were, or show any pictures of my old self. Obviously I was sharing my transformation on the internet. But I did not put it all out there as it actually was. I may never fully do that, as I feel no desire to peel the onions of my childhood and youth, which is where it all stemmed from. Now days as I look back & see things more clearly, I cannot believe that I had this weird kind of shame for not being genetically obese. I thought I do not deserve to inspire others with my pathetic story, when they have life much harder than I do. Or so I thought. Everyone has their own set of issues & demons they deal with. And

EVERYONE, myself included has the right and possibly even duty to inspire others with their own triumphs, victories, and achievements. I am still learning how to overcome these type of self - doubting thoughts. That is what is in my genetics. Self – doubt. Self – hate. Self – inflicted pain. The other 3 S's... It took me a very long time to allow myself to even think of myself as worthy of being an inspiration to others. Even when I was beaming with sun brightening aura & it seemed as if I had life by the tail. I always felt as if I was only worthy of inspiring ME – MYSELF - & I. Which that is not a bad thing in itself to be an inspiration for one's self. That is what we all should strive for. I had that part down. I just had decades of self – esteem, self – confidence issues that I needed to acknowledge if I ever was going to reach my full potential. It really wasn't that long ago when I started to address these issues I have & work on fixing them so that I can continue to level up on my own journey through life. I AM an inspiration to others. I AM a gift to the world. I Am worthy of happiness. I AM I AM... and guess what? You are as well. We all are interconnected to the Universe – whether we know it or not. At our core, we are divine spirits experiencing life through the lens of humanity. We may as well enjoy it - and encourage and inspire others to do the same.

I have something for you...

I am considering creating a public playlist on one of my YouTube channels specifically for this DLM Mastery Series. I am not 100% sure yet if I will do this, but if I do I would like to invite you to join in. I am also working on a private community to go along with an entire step by step DLM Mastery Course. This is all still in the works, so things are always subject to change. But I do want you to be in the know as there are at least more books I am working on in this specific series, and other related content that you may be interested in as well. Be sure to follow me on whatever platform you discovered this book from if they have the option. Many do. Also, follow me on **Instagram @dextersworld** & send me a message if you want to be on my list of people interested in the course or anything else that I have going on.

Carpe diem

DexRay

Hey, I thank you for spending this time with me.

If you got any time to quickly leave a review wherever it is that you discovered this book at I greatly appreciate that in advance! It means a lot to me & I do really enjoy reading them all, & appreciate every single one of you.

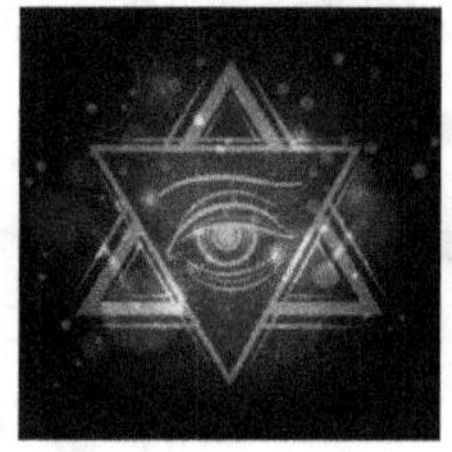

Disclaimer:

The content of this book is intended for informational and educational purposes only and is based on the author's personal experiences, theories, and interpretations. It is not intended as medical advice, diagnosis, or treatment. The information provided should not be used as a substitute for professional medical advice or guidance from a licensed healthcare provider.

Before making any changes to your diet, health regimen, or lifestyle, it is recommended to consult a qualified healthcare professional, especially if you have any existing health conditions, concerns, or dietary restrictions.

The author does not claim to offer cures or guarantees related to anti - aging, vitality, or spiritual practices discussed in this book. The reader assumes full responsibility for their own actions and choices.

Results may vary, and individual experiences may differ. The views expressed in this book are those of the author and do not necessarily reflect those of any medical or scientific authority.